WHEN PREGNANCY IS A PROBLEM

Regis Walling

ABBEY PRESS
St. Meinrad, Indiana 47577

Dedicated to
MARY AND ELIZABETH
who understand all the problems of
a "surprise" pregnancy
(Luke 1,2)

Second printing, 1985

PHOTO CREDITS: Mike Streff, Cover; Randy Dieter, page 4; Landrum B. Shettles, M.D., pages 12 and 13; Kay Freeman, page 50; Florence Sharp, page 92.

Library of Congress Catalog Card Number:
79-51280
ISBN: 0-87029-152-1

CONTENTS

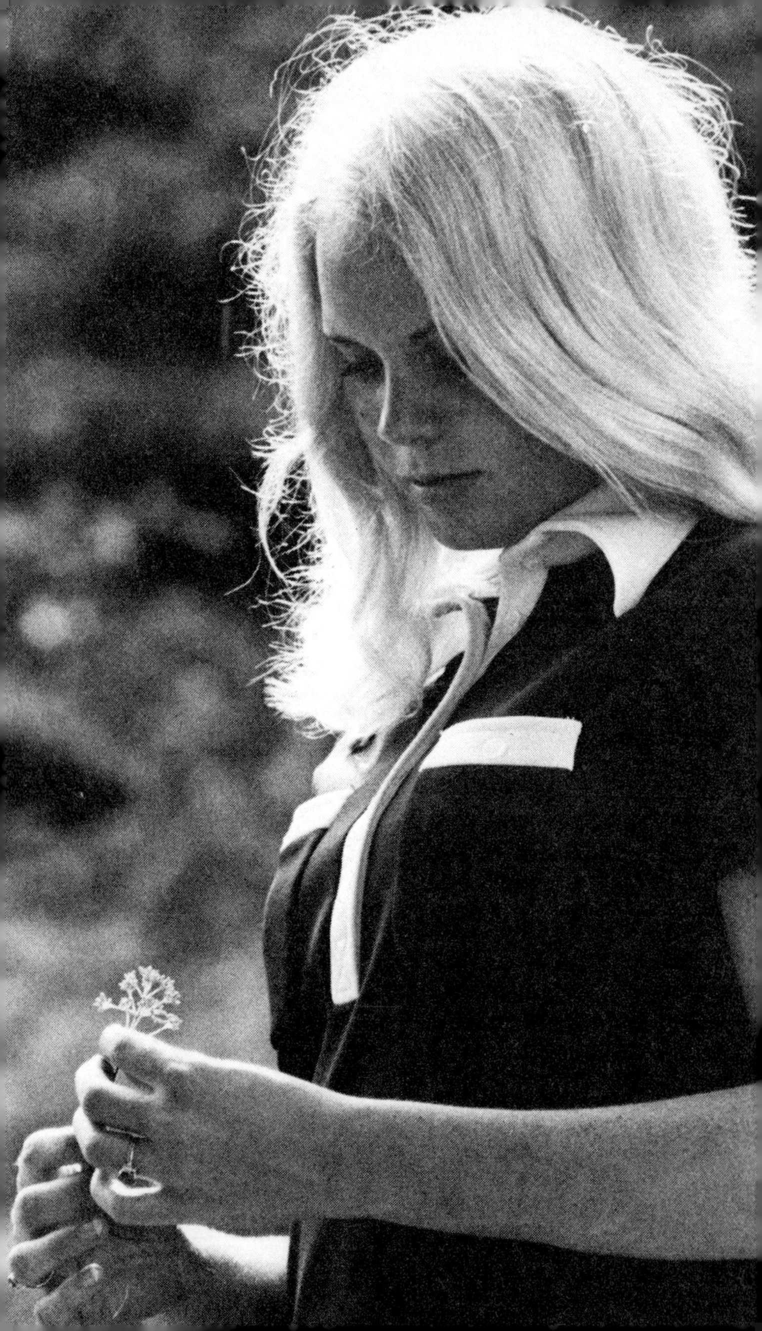

Preface

There are times when it is not good to be alone. The struggle to work through the dilemma of a difficult pregnancy is one of those times. Each of us has been "birthed" into life every time someone has cared about us. When pregnancy is a problem, it is the caring, understanding, and reaching out of others that can give the troubled, pregnant woman the inner strength to nurture and birth the child she is carrying.

There is scarcely a person whose family or circle of friends has not been touched by a pregnancy that was a problem. Such a pregnancy is often only a sign or a symptom of a more serious and deeper difficulty. Problems are personal and no two persons or sets of circumstances are the same. Love and care expressed to and for the pregnant woman will enable her to make the best decisions for all involved, including, in a special way, the baby.

Today when a pregnancy is a problem the first suggested solution is often abortion. In the musical, *Cabaret,* the singer, over the objection of her lover, aborts their child. Several scenes earlier she had received a cable from her father: he would not be coming for the long-awaited visit he had promised. Her disappointment and pain were obvious; her life had less love in it. Had she been "parented" by her father's visit, may she not have been able to parent the child within her?

My own experience in pregnancy counseling confirms that counselors are correct when they state that no woman can abort her child unless she herself has been psychologically aborted at some time in her life. Therefore, when someone suggests an abortion to you or for someone close to you, remember that the very suggestion is in itself an "abortion" and that loving and caring are the life-giving, "birthing" solutions.

Perhaps you have already had to cope with this problem. If you are like most of us, the first experience made you aware of your own need for much more thought and sensitivity and ready information. Some of that will be found in these pages. You will not find much statistical data, however, for two reasons. First, much of what is heard from professional workers, volunteers, and clients is not available in statistical form—such as the incidence of mental illness and suicide following an abortion or the increased level of abuse, physical and/or psychological toward other children that having an abortion can cause. Secondly, you are unique and your problem must have its own resolution.

It makes little difference if an outcome affects one in two women or one in ten thousand, if *you* are that one!

There are some observations that apply to everyone, and in the first and last chapters we will consider some of the common elements in the problem being faced, in the alternative solutions, and in the making of the decision. The middle chapters will offer some considerations for the particular situations of single and married women.

This book raises issues and questions. The answers, however, are for *you* to decide. Please discuss this information with a counselor, a trained volunteer, or with those who love you, especially your parents, a member of the clergy, or a teacher. If you need help in finding someone to talk to, you can call BIRTHRIGHT, toll free, 1-800-773-LOVE.

If you have had an abortion and need or want to talk about it and to understand and deal with your feelings, write to W.E.B.A. (Women Exploited By Abortion), P.O. Box 267, Schoolcraft, MI 49087.

The most important lessons we learn often come from our mistakes, from crises and from starting over. As difficult and untimely as your pregnancy may be, it may help you become a better, more mature, and more loving person. This, then, is my wish and prayer for you as you read and ponder these pages.

CHAPTER 1

Being Pregnant

Irene is nineteen. Nick is twenty-one. They are planning to be married in a year. Nick has a skill and a well-paying job. Irene is pregnant.

Susan and John have seven children. John has been unemployed on and off for six of the last eighteen months. Susan's health has not been good. She finds it most difficult to cope with her large family and to manage on their inadequate income. Susan and John are expecting their eighth child.

Carol is sixteen and Jack is eighteen. Although they really care about each other deeply, they both realize that neither is ready for marriage. Carol knows that she is not ready to care for the child she is carrying, and that her parents, at their age and with their other commitments, cannot accept the responsibility of caring for a new baby. Jack's parents prefer that Carol keep the baby and they promise financial help.

Ann and her husband have been married sixteen years. Ann is thirty-seven. They have four children; the youngest is ten. Ann feels that her family is at an age where she can resume her career as an interior decorator. She has taken courses to improve her skills and has found an opening with an established firm. She has just learned she is pregnant.

Peg is twenty-nine. She is seventeen weeks pregnant and has made several attempts to induce a miscarriage. Her question is "Where can I get an inexpensive abortion?"

Each of these people have the same problem—a pregnancy that was unplanned. None of them have the same problem pregnancy.

For Irene and Nick, considering their ages, his good job, and their intention of getting married, the problem is the timing of the pregnancy. The baby is, in fact, quite wanted and very welcome. Irene and Nick advance the date of their wedding. For them, marriage is the answer.

Susan and John are overwhelmed at the thought of another child to feed, clothe, and care for. The burdens of their situation are putting a real strain on their marriage relationship.

They are becoming hostile to each other.

In contrast, both Carol and Jack have good feelings about themselves. They can draw upon the support of their own inner resources and their understanding families. They are in regular contact with a counselor at a social services agency. They are making decisions based on a realistic assessment of their present abilities. Their primary concern is what is best for the baby. Carol and Jack decide that it is in the best interest of their child for them to release it for adoption.

When Ann learned she was pregnant she went into a period of deep depression and denial. Her self-confidence was shaken and old fears about her adequacy as an individual surfaced. She developed headaches and withdrew more and more into herself.

When she was seventeen Peg married. After four years of a very unhappy marriage her husband left her. As a child Peg was beaten by her mother; she has a history of drug and alcohol abuse, and has attempted suicide. Feeling completely broken after her divorce she "hit the bars" and paid for her drinks with sex. Out of such an encounter she became pregnant. The father of her now six-year-old son has disappeared.

In her utter desperation Peg is unable to think straight. She is trying to cope with her own loneliness, with a normal but also very lonely little boy, and with serious financial problems. She is seriously trying to find some sense of worth and purpose in herself.

These cases raise most of the crucial questions that accompany an unplanned pregnancy. Is the problem really the pregnancy itself? Or is the pregnancy symptomatic of deeper problems within the individual? What role do social circumstances and pressures play in the acceptance of a pregnancy? What immediate solutions are there? Which difficulties have only long-range answers? What is insoluble at the present time? Are there people or organizations which can help resolve the problems?

The initial panic and worry about an unplanned pregnancy, "What am I going to do?" lends itself to solution when broken down into smaller parts. Fortunately, nature provides nine months to prepare for the birth of a baby.

The People Involved

There are a number of persons whom being pregnant affects. Each person is extremely important and has rights and feelings which must be respected. Most of this book is directed to the pregnant mother, but first we will briefly consider the others whose lives are affected.

The Baby

The tiniest but most important person is the unborn child. From the eighteenth day after conception the baby's heart has been beating. By the eighth week, only two weeks after the mother's second missed period, the son or

Prenatal Development

Age of Unborn	Development	Size
18-25 days	Heart begins to beat	1/8 inch
6 weeks	Brain waves recordable Nerves and muscles formed Skeleton completed and moves All body parts present	½ inch
7 weeks	Nerves and muscles coordinated Stomach produces gastric juices Liver makes blood Kidneys purify blood Sex organs visible All 20 milk-teeth buds present	5/8 inch 1/30 ounce
8 weeks (2 months)	Brain completely present Active arm and leg movements Permanent fingerprints	1 inch
9-10 weeks	Sex hormones identifiable Glands function Squints, swallows, moves tongue Wakes and sleeps	1 ¾ inches

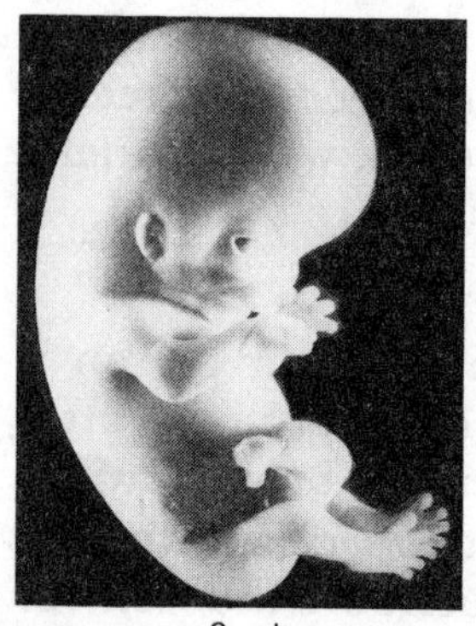

8 wks.

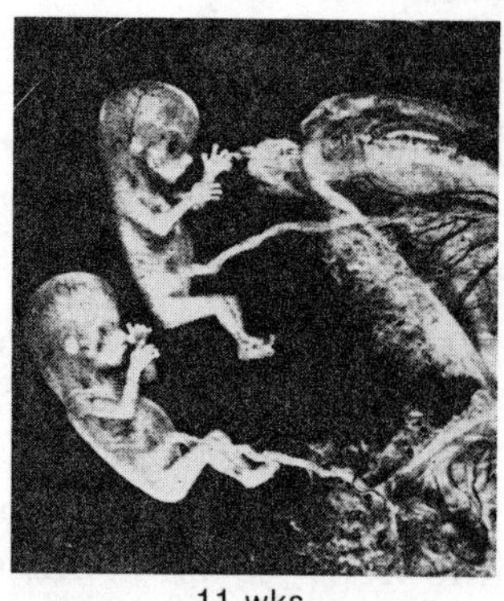

11 wks.

Age of Unborn	Development	Size
11-12 weeks (3 months)	All body parts functioning Sucks thumb; hiccups Refined arm and leg movements Begins ''breathing''fluid Fingernails formed Psychological traits being developed	3 inches 1 ounce
16 weeks (4 months)	Eyelashes formed Nose, lips, and ears complete	5-6 inches 4-6 ounces
5 months	Hair grows	10-12 inches ½-1 pound
6 months	Eyelids separated	11-14 inches 1 ¼-1 ½ lbs.
7 months	Eyes open	14-17 inches 2 ½-3 lbs.
8 months	Maturation	16-19 inches 4 ½-5 ½ lbs.
9 months	Birth	Average 20 inches; 7 lbs.

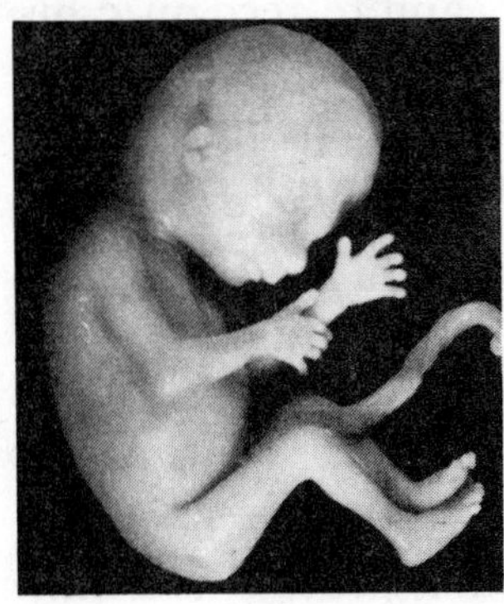

16 wks.

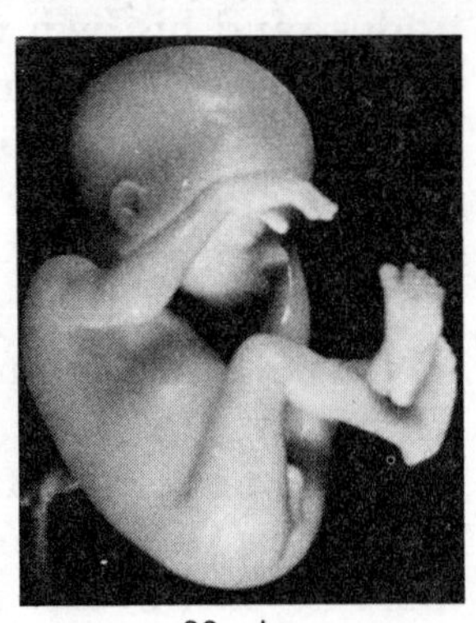

20 wks.

daughter is fully formed, and now needs only time and nourishment for continued growth and development. The baby is so small that its motion cannot be felt even though intrauterine and sonal photography show that it is already moving its hands and feet and is bouncing around in the amniotic fluid. The baby is adjusting to the mother's schedule, to her activity, to her moods, and is well on its way to developing its own basic personality. The above chart and photos illustrate the development of the baby.

The Father

The father of the baby is important not just for conception but to the total pregnancy. Though it is true that some men will not stand by their wives or girl friends, it is also a fact that many will *if* they are brought into the counseling and decision-making process regarding the unplanned pregnancy. Unless he is helped to understand his own values and to recognize his own feelings, a man may develop a negative self-image or seek to cover his emotions by escaping into more sexual activity with new partners (or into alcohol, drugs, or other self-defeating behaviors).

The father's ambivalence is in part a reflection of the legal contradictions facing him —he has no right whatever to protect the life of his unborn baby, but, if the child is born, he must be part of any adoption process and may be liable financially for the baby.* It is to his advantage, to the mother's, and ultimately to the baby's, if the father takes part in the counseling.

Occasionally, and often through no fault of his own, the father knows little about pregnancy and the development of the baby. One college student abruptly left a class during a film depicting early prenatal development. The professor found him in the corridor, sobbing bitterly. All that he could say was "I didn't know it was a baby! I would never have paid for it (an abortion) if I had known!" This young man needed intensive counseling for nearly a year to be able to face daily life without a crippling sense of guilt.

The Family

When a woman announces an unplanned pregnancy, her family may react in a variety of ways. Caring parents (or a loving spouse) may experience great pain and disappointment because they have dreamed of her happiness. Their hurt may initially manifest itself as anger at the mother-to-be, at the boy friend, at *themselves* because they feel they have failed. The pregnant woman and the family, however, can and must help each other. There are many problems to be resolved and each person involved needs his or her psychic energy. Why

*Because state laws vary the father should consult a social worker to understand both his rights and his responsibilities.

waste it on blame and resentment that does nothing to contribute to positive feelings or solutions?

After the announcement of the pregnancy but before any discussion or attempts at resolution, each person involved could profit from some *quiet time* and *separate space* to think through the emotions of the others. Each needs to clarify and to acknowledge his or her own deepest feelings. *Then,* calmly and gently, each will be able to share with the others what is really going on at an intellectual and at a feeling level. The emphasis must be on really *listening,* not only to the words, but more, to the feelings, the dreams—to what is unsaid between the words. Each should keep in mind that:

Others have survived and grown through similar experiences.

A mistake in loving is *not* the worst thing a person might do.

Every life history contains wrong choices and unpleasant memories.

We do not need perfect parents, spouses, or children. We do need to be human. Coping with hurt and failure is a human task.

Because pregnancy is so visible it calls for greater solidarity and support within the family.

This is a time to forgive with love and to love with forgiveness—for the past and in the present.

Each person can choose whether this crisis will be a time of disintegration or an occasion for renewed love and caring. It is not what we go through but what we grow through that counts.

You

Are you really pregnant? Have you had a pregnancy test *and* a pelvic examination to be sure that, if you are pregnant, the baby is in the uterus and not in a Fallopian tube. If you do not have money or you fear going to a doctor who knows you (and your family), contact your local Birthright or similar organization and a trained volunteer will help you make arrangements. You may go to your local public health service, but be aware that at some public clinics some staff members may attempt to pressure you to abort. There are so-called Women's or Feminist Health Centers that offer *free* pregnancy tests. However, these are often inaccurate and they are usually free *only* if you agree to abort if the results are positive.

While awaiting the results of your pregnancy test, you may wish to re-examine your goals, values, and friendships. Are they what you want them to be? Do they make your life happy and satisfying? Should the pregnancy test prove negative, you may still discover that you want to change some of the directions of your life. Anyone who could assist you in coping with pregnancy will also be glad to talk with you about these other matters.

If the results of your pregnancy test are positive and you are afraid to tell your parents, boyfriend, or husband, an in-between step may be a conference with a trained volunteer or social worker. This person can help you to get in touch with your feelings and to analyze your situation, and can explain what you need to know about pregnancy, birth, *all* the consequences of abortion, and the services that are available to you in your community. This information will make you more sure of yourself. You may even practice how you might tell others. This worker may well become a friend who will help you and your family throughout the entire crisis, and beyond.

If you are pregnant there are many reasons why you can feel good about yourself. *Because* you are in crisis, you have an opportunity to remake or to redirect your life. Even more, you can marvel at the *wonder* of new life that is forming within you. You have been entrusted with a unique, never-to-be-repeated-in-the-whole-history-of-the-world life. It is a "wonder-full" thing that has happened.

The very fact that you are reading this book says that you are admitting your limitations, that you are seeking information, and that you want to make a responsible decision. You have courage or by now you would have taken the "easy way out." Your courage is there to be used, one step at a time.

The first reaction of a social worker or a

volunteer to a call from you will be a recognition of your strength and of your willpower, for everyone in a helping position knows how very difficult it is to ask for another's help, especially in a situation such as this.

At times the person whom it is most difficult to face in total honesty is *oneself*. Facing yourself not on a superficial level but at the very core of your being can convince you that you have value simply because you exist. Success or failure, right decisions or mistakes, good actions or bad—nothing changes your intrinsic worth as a person. If anyone thinks less of you, that is that person's problem—it may hurt you, deeply, but it can change you *only* if *you* let it affect you.

Understanding the Causes

As you attempt to work through your feelings about your pregnancy the important question is not "Why did I get pregnant?" but rather "Why did I have intercourse?"

Was it the first time? It makes quite a difference if this was the only occasion (or if you have had intercourse a few times but at widely spaced intervals) rather than part of a general pattern of behavior. Furthermore, if you have had only one partner you differ from a person who has had several or many "lovers." Was it a fully conscious choice or was any alcohol or drug use involved? Did you consent willingly or reluctantly? Was it because you wanted to experiment to see what "sex" was like or do (did) you really love him? These are difficult questions, but they must be faced if you are to come to grips with your life.

Perhaps there were some subconscious dynamics operating. Were you trying to keep your boyfriend's affection? When a woman is very lonely she may mistake a man's interest as being deeper than it really is.

Everyone has "skin hungers" but in some families affection is seldom expressed or, if it is shown, it is by word only and not by hugs or touching. When people have not learned that there are many nonerotic ways of touching, they may conclude that intercourse is necessary to show deep warmth or to communicate real affection. Is this what happened to you?

Or have you been experiencing turmoil in other parts of your life? "Sex" can be used as an escape from family expectations or from school pressures. At times it can be a means of getting revenge against parents or against a previous boyfriend. It may also be a price for being part of a certain "in" group.

Genital activity and pregnancy may also be a means of getting attention. One young woman from a prominent and wealthy family had her fourth pregnancy when she was nineteen years old. The only time that her parents seemed to know that she was alive was when she was pregnant. Possibly on a subconscious level you hoped to become pregnant so that someone would notice you. Perhaps you wanted someone to love, and who, in turn, would love you. Maybe you have had so much inner pain that this became a way for you to cry out for help.

How you respond to these questions will help you to discern the real issues which you must confront. If the questions are ignored, you will very likely have a repeat crisis pregnancy.

You have to deal with two parallel and critical situations—the resolution of the pregnancy itself *and* the resolution of those basic needs which are the source of the pregnancy.

Society

The same society which has created the atmosphere which made it easy for you to get into this situation may well condemn you for "getting caught." Society today offers you an abortion as a solution. There is the implication that if you do not abort this unwanted pregnancy you will end up physically and psychologically abusing your child. The abortionists ignore all the evidence and statistics which prove that it is parents who were abused themselves as children or those who wanted a child for their own ego-satisfaction that tend to exploit or injure their offspring. However, you will do well to keep each of these points in mind when you are making your decision about whether you will marry, raise the child as a single parent, or will release the baby for adoption.

Should you abort your baby and should

you succeed in hiding the fact from everyone else, *you* will always have the experience as one of *your* memories. There is no such thing as a "safe" abortion. Whether they are physical or psychological, immediate or delayed, the consequences of abortion are part of a woman's life as long as she lives.

In six years in pregnancy counseling work, I never met a woman who had aborted and who had no negative results. In contrast, I have encountered many instances of women in their sixties and seventies and even in their eighties who are literally tortured by an abortion undergone long ago.

Among women having abortions today, the scars become visible in depression, in a lower self-image, and in guilt feelings (which are more often psychological than religious). Something happens to a person when that person is responsible for ending a human life, whatever the circumstances.

Abortion is particularly destructive to one's sense of personal self-worth. Having an abortion reinforces a sense of not being worth noticing or caring about. Psychologists are reporting that among those women having an abortion, marriage relationships are harmed and often broken, and abuse to any other children increases. There is a tendency to marry or to associate with a spouse abuser and there is a greater readiness to resort to violence to solve other social problems by those who abort or who advocate abortion.

Since an abortion is an indication of the woman's failure to deal with the issues behind the pregnancy, there is a high incidence of second unwanted pregnancies following an abortion.

Physical complications from abortion are very real. Miscarriages occur more frequently among women who have had an abortion. Abortion can also cause sterility.

Society offers a variety of assistance to those in need of temporary help and these are available to you in your pregnancy. At the same time you will feel the pressure of society to abort rather than use these services; you will be made to feel guilty if you accept public assistance. National figures may correlate with the Michigan experience that if you do receive financial aid to help with the costs of prenatal care, delivery, and the days immediately following the birth, you will be off the public roll in less time than the woman who has a state-paid abortion. Further, the same evidence proves that, if you do not have an abortion, you are less apt to need help again because you will have put your life into focus.

Understanding Pregnancy

Pregnancy affects your total self, your body, emotions, and spirit. Understanding the full meaning of being pregnant can help you when pregnancy is a problem.

The Beginning Stages

As soon as the sperm fertilizes the ovum, changes begin to occur in your entire body. Every cell and hormone mobilizes for the protection and growth of this new life. The uterine lining is prepared for implantation, your breasts swell and become tender because of hormone changes and because the water content of your body increases. Your cervix lifts and becomes firm, and you *know* that something is happening! These changes may cause nausea or "morning sickness" and you may crave certain foods or resist others. Each of the changes is a sign of health, just as pregnancy itself is a *healthy* condition. Physical problems that do occur during this time have other causes and should be given medical attention. If you are not sure that something is normal during pregnancy, call the matter to the attention of your doctor *immediately*!

The hormone changes trigger emotional changes. The normal pregnancy cycle brings with it depression, often severe, from about the eighth to the fourteenth week. The future seems hopeless, every fear becomes magnified, and suspicion and edginess work their way into nearly every encounter. These feelings come even in a pregnancy that is wanted and planned. Because of this depression, no major life-changing decisions of any kind should be made during these weeks.

Diet and Exercise

A diet that is good for your general health, weight control, and complexion is also what you need during pregnancy. Protein (milk, eggs, cheese, meat) and fresh fruits and vegetables are basic to feeling fit and energetic. It is essential for the health of your baby and for your future pregnancies that you give careful attention to your diet.

Fats and salty foods may cause a retention of fluids and an excessive weight gain that will make your pregnancy more uncomfortable. If you are taking any kind of drugs, including over-the-counter medication such as aspirin, or any chemical, such as alcohol, you should stop immediately as some of these substances may pass through to the baby. Should you have a prescription, it is prudent to call your doctor or to ask your pharmacist if the medicine could affect your unborn child.

A continuous supply of oxygen is critical for your baby, especially during the first weeks of its development when the vital organs, particularly its brain, are being formed. If you smoke, carbon monoxide replaces some of the oxygen in your own blood and not only is the supply of good oxygen for your baby impeded but the carbon monoxide can pass through the placenta and do real harm. If you cannot stop smoking completely it is advisable that you lessen as much as possible the amount you smoke.

The formation of the baby's bones requires calcium. In addition to milk being necessary in your diet for the baby, it is also important for your own dental hygiene. Try to see your dentist at least once during your pregnancy; the earlier you do so the better it will be for your own well-being and comfort.

How much do you exercise daily? The more you keep your muscles loose by regular activity, especially by brisk walking, the better overall tone and good feeling your body will have. You'll sleep more soundly and, when the time comes, have an easier labor and delivery.

From the Fourteenth Week on

From about the fourteenth week through the seventh month you will experience, in varying degrees, a sense of wholeness and well-being. The morning nausea will disappear and many women report that at this time they feel "great!" Toward the end of the pregnancy your feelings will be mixed. You may have trouble sleeping and so be very tired and uncomfortable. At the same time, you will start to get impatient for the baby's birth and yet be a bit apprehensive as you anticipate labor and delivery. All of this is normal unless there are other health problems complicating the process.

Coping with the Pregnancy

In coping with an unplanned pregnancy, it helps to break the problem down into smaller parts. You might use a form similar to the sample on page 28. Note that some questions occur at certain times and others remain. For example, the question of meeting medical expenses could be a matter to be dealt with throughout the pregnancy. Some problems have no answers. The important thing is to surface each question that is part of the overall problem and to settle upon a response. After studying the sample you might work with the blank form on page 29. You can add to it or subtract from it as your pregnancy progresses.

There really is no "good time" to be pregnant or to have a baby. In spite of this, your pregnancy does not have to interrupt your schedule completely nor should it cause you to change all your plans.

One reason for taking care of your general health during pregnancy is that you may continue your regular activities until close to your time of delivery. Some women have been able to continue working until a few days before the birth of the baby. It is more prudent, however, to take some time off before the baby comes. If you are well rested, labor will be easier. Remember that the baby will keep you from getting a full night's sleep for some time after its birth.

It might be helpful to list in chronological order everything you have planned for the months ahead. Then attempt to forecast how being pregnant will affect you in doing all you

Sample Problems	Now	Before Birth	After Birth	No Answer	Course of Action
Pregnancy					
Bad timing—family's vacation planned	x				Change place or activity
Sense of shame, guilt	x				Talk it out
Rh factor		x			Seek medical information
Fear of telling	x				Use a third party
Reaction of younger brothers/sisters		x			Investigate alternate housing
Baby					
Not ready to settle down	x		x		Face reality; growth will come
Fear of labor and delivery		x			Childbirth classes
Can't support a baby	x		x		Job placement; vocational education
Circumstances					
Boyfriend an alcoholic	x			x	Join Al-Anon; urge him to join AA
Abused as child	x				Find a counselor
Your age	x	x	x		Analyze inner strength; build support system

Your Problems	Now	Before Birth	After Birth	No Answer	Course of Action
Pregnancy					
Baby					
Circumstances					

Sample: High school senior, 2 months pregnant at beginning of Feb.

Month	Activity	OK as planned	Do in alternate way	Do later	Cancel
F 3	School	x			
	Future Nurses	x			
	Work evenings	x			
M 4	School	x			
	Future Nurses	x			
	Work evenings	x			
	Ping-Pong tourney	x			
A 5	School	x			
	Easter trip with classmates	?			? $
	Future Nurses	x			
	Begin ballet				x
	Work evenings	x			
M 6	School		x		
	Senior prom	?			
	Work evenings	?			
J 7	Exams	x			
	Graduation	Depends on school policy/ personal choice			
	Vacation trip	?			? $
J 8	Tennis tourney				x
A 9	Work evenings				x
S 10	Start college	Will depend on whether you keep the baby or release it for adoption			
O 11	College				

Month	Your Projected Activities and Timetable	OK as planned	Do in alternate way	Do later	Cancel

have planned. Some of your plans, depending on how you feel and how big you grow, may have to be changed. See the sample chart on page 30 and then use the blank form on page 31 to make your plans.

Medical Problems

The presence of the Rh factor, diabetes, a heart problem, or another chronic condition can complicate a pregnancy. Today, however, there are technologies that can prevail over most physical handicaps and ailments.

You may have reason to fear the birth of a mentally or physically impaired child. With counseling, you can work through these fears and learn of the many programs which can help such a person to achieve his or her full potential. The problem of handicapped people lies with so-called "normal" people, who judge the value of handicapped lives out of their own limited frame of reference.

Recently, Marjorie Guthrie, widow of composer-singer Woody Guthrie whose death at the age of forty resulted from Huntington's Disease (a hereditary condition), noted how poor the world would be without the richness of Woody's music. One suspects that Arlo Guthrie is also glad that his father lived.

In *The Terrible Choice* Pearl Buck testifies to the comfort and practical help that her own severely retarded daughter gave to others, showing that even though she is gravely retarded her life is most worthwhile.

Suicide seldom occurs among the handicapped. Perhaps their suffering has taught them that life is precious in itself, and does not depend on someone else's standard of "perfection" or on being "wanted."

However, there are many valid reasons why some families cannot care for an impaired child. Fortunately, there are foster and adoptive homes waiting for such children if the natural family cannot cope with the burden.

The suitable resolution of a crisis pregnancy, as we have seen, takes into account the woman who is pregnant and everyone who touches her life. It considers the causes which led to the pregnancy as well as those problems specific to it. In other words, the pregnancy is merely one part of a total situation and it is self-defeating to consider it in isolation.

In several significant respects, the problems of the unmarried woman vary from those of one who has a husband. These are our next considerations.

CHAPTER 2
The Unmarried Woman

The unmarried women considered in this chapter are the women who have careers, those who are college students, and those who are still minors, whether or not they are now in school.

You, a Career Woman

If you are a single career woman who learns she is pregnant, you must decide whether your *ultimate vocational goals* are compatible with raising a child. This is true whether you are firmly established in a lifework or just entering the professional world.

You may have planned to pursue a career or profession for a limited time prior to marriage and raising a family. If so, the problem is the timing of the pregnancy. Is the man involved your intended husband? If so, how has he reacted to the pregnancy and to the possibility of advancing your wedding date?

If the baby's father is not the person you would marry, how do you think the man whom you hope to eventually marry will respond to raising another man's child?

If these questions bring negative responses, you should seriously consider releasing the baby for adoption.

There is the possibility that neither your work nor your marriage plans included children. In this case to release the child for adoption would be the alternative *least* disruptive to your designs. Otherwise, the presence and needs of the baby will limit your availability for business travel, will certainly curtail your social life, will make further career education unlikely, and will lessen the overall chances for career advancement. You will almost inevitably become resentful towards the baby which would be damaging to both the life of the child and your own life. Frequently, when a career woman keeps her baby, there are no additional children and the child faces the loneliness of being an "only child."

Regardless of what you decide about the future of your baby you will almost certainly have to handle the emotional strain caused by the judgmental attitudes of some of your co-workers. This is particularly true if the father of your baby is a co-worker and if this fact is general knowledge. You may have to consider transferring to another work environment, especially if the company or organization is relatively small. Whether it was one mistake or a series of encounters that led to your pregnancy, even so-called "liberated" people tend to pigeonhole and to scorn the woman who "got caught." Unfortunately, it will be a long time before such attitudes die.

You may experience injustices in matters of health benefits, working days and hours, and/or promotions. You might have to use the avenues of legal redress that are open to you.

This is for you a critical time, a time for reflection and reevaluating your choice of a direction for your life. A counselor or social worker as a neutral and objective "outsider" could be your greatest help.

You, a College Woman

As a pregnant college student, you have to clarify your life goal in much the same way as does a career woman. What do you really want for your life?

It is not unusual for a woman to enter college with a very general goal and with the hope of discovering a program that will interest her as a life choice. Other students may begin college with well-defined objectives and a timetable for achieving them. Regardless of how firm your plans for the future have been up to this point, this pregnancy has made it necessary for you to decide now what you really do want. Your pregnancy may cause a temporary adjustment of your timetable, but it does not have to change your basic plans.

Your relationship to the baby's father must be carefully evaluated. The possibility of marriage must be considered in the same manner as suggested for the career woman. There may be an additional complication if the father and/or future husband is also still studying. What adjustments will marriage cause in his educational planning? How will it change his current financial status? Counseling for *both* of you could help you to understand your true feelings and hopes for your joint and individual futures. Seek guidance so that whatever changes you both do make will not swell into future bitterness.

There is the probability that you may want to continue your own education as far as possible. If you are healthy, there is probably no reason why you cannot complete the current semester. Your advisor or a school counselor can help you to plan for the time immediately before and after the birth of the baby. You might consider home study courses to maintain your class standing.

Your exploration of the reasons why you had intercourse may have revealed a subconscious attempt to find a way out of school. Have you lost interest in your studies? Are you satisfied with your grades? Did you come to a requirement which seemed to be beyond your capabilities? Perhaps there are some nonacademic circumstances feeding your dissatisfaction. Are you away from home and feeling lonely? Does your dormitory or apartment living satisfy your needs? How do you relate to your roommate—do you share values, ideas, interests, and life-style? How is she reacting to you and to your pregnancy? If she is not supportive, you may have to arrange for another living situation.

Some colleges and universities have health facilities on the campus. Be sure to investigate these and all other student benefits available to you. At the same time, consult a social services program off campus and explore the assistance available to you through these other groups. Many such services both on and off campus will attempt to counsel you to an abortion. Find out in advance how your potential counselor stands on abortion. Birthright, Lifeline, or a similar organization is always available to help you find what is best for both you and the baby.

Above all, if it is possible, try to include your parents in your deliberations, at least to the extent that you let them know what is happening. They should hear it from you, and not from an outsider. Depending on *how* you present it to them, this crisis could evolve into a positive means of cementing your adult friendship with them.

You, an Adolescent

Throughout history and in many cultures in our time, a woman who has matured physically is accepted as an adult. Marriage occurs and childbearing begins. It is only a recent development in the industrialized world, with its availability of universal education, that adulthood has been postponed, creating that period of time known as adolescence. This is an interval between physical maturity and the legal, cultural, and economic ability to be responsible for the consequences of adult sexual activity.

Regarding this interim there are two distinct and opposed schools of thought. One group would encourage the postponement of genital activity until the person is capable of coping with the consequences, physical, psychological, and economic, in the real world today. The opposition advocates full "freedom" for youth to engage in sexual acts, denies that any psychological harm can occur because of such split-level emotional living, and would simply "eliminate" any "unwanted consequence" that follows.

You, the teenaged person, are caught in the middle, hearing "Yes" and "No" at the same time, and now, if you are pregnant, you know the strong and conflicting pressures.

First of all, *you need to hear again that pregnancy is a normal, healthy condition.* You do not have a "sexually transmitted disease" nor are you part of some contagious "epidemic," so you do not need to be isolated or quarantined.

It is a fact, though, that babies born to teenage mothers do tend to have a lower birth-weight. They are more often born prematurely and are thus subject to the results of prematurity, such as retardation. The reason for these problems is not so much the age of the mother, as the frequently inadequate American teenage diet. Most of the baby's formation has been completed by the time the doctor confirms the pregnancy, so that, unless an adolescent woman has generally good nutrition habits, some developmental deficiencies are possible.

Fear often prevents a young woman from getting early prenatal care. Such care would prevent most problems in pregnancy from becoming serious for the mother and potentially dangerous for the baby. This is a plea to any woman, of any age, reading these pages to make a habit of good nutrition, to maintain a regular exercise pattern, and if she suspects a pregnancy to see a doctor immediately. Proper care can eliminate much prematurity and the problem of low birth-weight of infants born to young women.

Second, *you have a decision to make on the future of your baby*. You may choose to place the baby for adoption, to marry the child's father, to marry your intended husband who may not be the child's father, to raise the baby as a single parent, or to have your parents raise the child within your family. There are those who will attempt to persuade you to consider abortion as an option. There are some facts about abortion you should know.

Abortion of a first pregnancy and especially by a young mother can jeopardize *all* her future children (if this abortion does not cause sterility). In the course of a pregnancy and labor, the cervical muscle gradually strengthens and enlarges so that the baby can be delivered. In abortion the cervix is dilated (stretched) by force before the natural elasticity can develop. In a manner similar to a rubber band that is stretched too far, the cervix loses some of its strength so that it may become too weak to hold the weight of a future, full-term baby. The woman who aborts her first pregnancy is greatly adding to the chances against her *ever* carrying a baby for nine months.

You should ponder the fact that evidence indicates that all women who abort experience long-term and profound grief. Occasionally an older woman is able to deny these feelings and to bury them (and they do their damage from within). The young woman, on the other hand, is more apt to have these feelings very intensely and openly. Pregnancy counselors report an increasing number of "atonement" pregnancies in which the woman becomes pregnant expressly to replace the baby she aborted.

Finally, *you must know that the law places the total power of choice over your baby into your hands.* Legally, no one can force you to abort. If anyone should try to coerce you to end your baby's life, you can call *any* law officer and ask to be placed "in protective custody." Both you and your baby will be safe.

In choosing to carry your baby to birth, you are making a choice of which you can be proud. You will always know that you succeeded when it was very difficult, and whether you keep your baby or place it for adoption, you can be pleased with your growing courage and maturity.

An Open Letter to Your Parents

Dear Parents,

Your teenage daughter is going to be a parent. This is *your* child and your grandchild—you cannot be neutral on-lookers.

Basically, you have only two alternatives. You can respond with caring love, be understanding and supportive, and help your daughter make positive choices toward rebuilding and redirecting her life, or you can respond negatively and destructively.

An out-of-wedlock pregnancy is not the worst catastrophe that could happen. Parents of adolescents who have died of drug overdose, auto accident, or suicide will tell you to be glad that your teen is still alive. Parents of young people who are imprisoned would say that you should be thankful your teen has no record, and parents whose children have run away would remind you that you do have your daughter with you.

Those of us who have counseled adolescents will assure you that "bad" teens do not become pregnant—they planned to have intercourse and "took precautions." It is the basically good young person for whom the situation got out of hand that becomes pregnant.

We also remind you that all of us have those things in our past of which we are not proud, and they may be much more serious but less *visible* than an unwed pregnancy. If you can keep this problem in perspective you will have a good beginning for dealing with it.

A pregnancy, like most other family events, is complex and affects everyone in the family. It is extremely important that you now show concern for your daughter as a person and not just for the pregnancy which will last only a few months.

Your recognition that this crisis is a family difficulty should make it easier for you to become a part of the counseling process *if* your concern is truly for how you can help your daughter. Parents who fear or refuse to participate in family counseling usually cannot face and deal with their own personal problems or with their own marital relationship that needs attention and healing.

To agree to participate in the counseling process is an effective way of assuring your daughter that you are with her, that you do love her for herself, and that even a serious mistake cannot destroy your love.

If you attempt to pressure her to have an

abortion, you will be telling her that what family and friends may say if she delivers the baby is more important to you than she is. You are telling her that her physical and psychologial wellbeing do not matter to you. You are implying that she is not good enough or mature enough to learn from her mistake. And, finally, you are indicating that it is acceptable to destroy a human life rather than to accept the responsibility for one's own personal actions. She will have little reason to look up to you anymore. You will have paid a high price—the sacrifice of your chances for a future adult friendship with her.

Mother, how much is your daughter like you? One reason a young woman rebels is precisely because she is like her mother and is trying to discover her own unique identity. You can help to bridge the gap between you if you can remember back to your own first loves and to your feelings and fears during your first pregnancy. As women, you have much now which you can discuss and share. To accept her as an adult and to encourage her adult responsibility will foster that adult friendship which will enrich both of your lives.

Dad, do you still think of this daughter as "your little girl"? Didn't you notice how she has become a young woman—how she now resembles the woman with whom you fell in love and married? Perhaps that is why you have felt so hurt and so angry with the boy who "did this" to her. But, Dad, you were fortunate that you grew up at a time when a fellow had more encouragement to be in control of his feelings, no matter how strong they were. At least you can credit both of these young people with sincerity and attempt to understand their feelings. They need you now to help them face the realities of their situation. Your support is critical to the decisions your daughter must make.

There is one lesson which every human being needs to learn, and which *you* in particular can teach: there is a loving Father who understands each person, forgives each failing, and who loves us eternally.

Mom and Dad, as an adolescent your daughter wavers between being an adult and being a child. You face the challenge to be fully adult in this crisis—to recognize your feelings and keep them under control, to be conscious of your values and the reasons for your beliefs, and to be rational and calm in each discussion. To the extent that you treat your daughter as an adult, you will help her to achieve the maturity she needs to rebuild her life when the pregnancy is over and the child is born.

All of this is a tremendous challenge, but there are many who would help you meet the challenge. Reach out to help and be helped.

Best wishes,

Incest and Rape

Because the victims of incest and rape are

usually young and unmarried, they are included in this chapter. These observations, however, apply to each situation regardless of the age and marital status of the victim.

Along with the legalized violence against the helpless unborn, the last decade has witnessed a great increase in all forms of brutality—frightful weaponry, crime, child and spouse abuse. Incest and rape are two manifestations of this same vicious disregard for innocent life.

Both incest and rape have been part of the long history of the exploitation of women. The victims of these crimes have suffered alone and in silence for much too long. Each of these attacks is a devastating occurrence for the victim who needs the kind of help that will not do *further violence,* physical or psychological, to her. The reaction, that if a pregnancy does result from either cause the woman ought to have an abortion, really says that she should pay the long-term price for the act of which she is a victim.

There is, in one sense, no reason for surprise at the increase of both incest and rape. The contraceptive mentality has taught the lessons that a woman should always "be ready" and that a man should never "have to wait." The result is that many women and children will have life-long scars from the traumas of incest and rape.

In public debate, rape and incest are usually linked together even though they are different in significant ways and each deserves individual consideration.

Incest

Perhaps the strongest taboo that society has is that against incest. As a result, although episodes of incest are much more common today than ever before, the taboo works against both the victim who fears to report it, and the incestuous man who, even if he wants to, is usually too ashamed to admit his need for help. Because incest is happening so much more often, *every* person to whom a child reports being molested must take the child seriously and pursue appropriate action immediately.

Reporting the act to the authorities should be done for the victim's sake, as well as for the sake of the one committing incest. In a very high percentage of cases those committing incest can be helped through counseling and other forms of therapy.

The victim needs a great deal of assurance that she (or he) is not "bad" or "dirty," that she did right in telling, that she is safe and will not be harmed. It may be necessary, at least temporarily, that the victim be placed in protective custody or that another place to live be found.

The child has quite likely been threatened. An older child has probably been told to "keep quiet or I'll have to do this with your sister/s (and brother/s)." If such a threat is reported, the other persons are usually *already* being abused and need to be reached and helped.

In the few instances in which pregnancy does occur through incest, the woman especially needs long-term intensive help. The baby is, in fact, less a problem than the psychological aftermath of the incestuous act. No matter how a pregnancy begins, birth is still safer than abortion for a woman. However, because of the circumstances, this baby is one who really should be released for adoption.

Rape

In contrast to incest which is sexual aggression against a family member, rape is most often a violent crime of power against a weak and unknown person. The woman who is raped should go or be taken immediately to a hospital for medical treatment, and should also report the rape immediately to the police. Today the rape victim has access to special crisis workers, and the trauma does not have to destroy her.

Pregnancy from rape is very rare, yet it can happen. There is no way, however, that subjecting the woman to the second trauma of abortion can eliminate the traumatic experience of the rape from her life. In this instance, too, adoption is most probably the best decision.

In my own counseling experience, women who indicated that they had become pregnant by forced intercourse (by rape or by drunken or coercive husbands) and who gave birth to the baby were unanimous in their certainty that they had decided rightly. How many persons who are part of our daily lives were conceived unwillingly we will never know. Regardless of how a child is conceived, he or she is a gift to us all.

Throughout the pregnancy that does result from rape the woman deserves a great deal of supportive caring, counseling, and help in affirming her positive self-image and future life. Compassion is a powerful factor in healing this wound.

Whatever her age or situation and whatever the cause of the pregnancy, the unmarried woman has need of much supportive concern from her family and from everyone else whom she encounters. Her future lies ahead of her and need not be determined by her past.

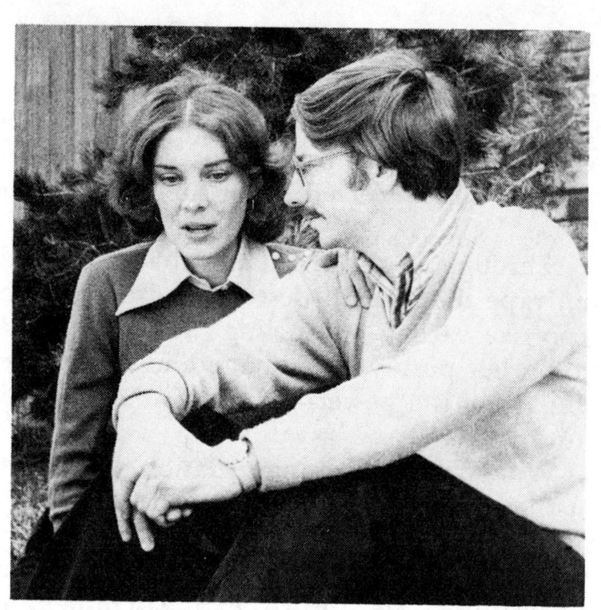

CHAPTER 3
The Married Woman

One day the second grade teacher had each child tell a "happy thought" to the other students. She came to one little girl who smiled sweetly and announced, "I'm pregnant!" Although quite surprised, the teacher quickly went on to the next pupil. Later in the day she had a chance to speak to the child.

"Now, dear," she asked, "what was that happy thought you told us this morning?"

"I'm pregnant," the girl repeated.

"And why is that your happy thought today?" continued the teacher.

"Well," the girl answered, "when Daddy came down to breakfast this morning my Mommy told him 'Honey, I think I'm pregnant' and he said 'Isn't that a happy thought!' "

Whether or not it is a "happy thought" your pregnancy is a fact. That you are reading this book is an indication that this pregnancy is not a completely happy thought. Your concern may arise from a number of circumstances, all aggravated by your depressed mood which is normal in early pregnancy. There is probably no woman who, however much she has wanted a baby, would not prefer to avoid the pregnancy and labor part of the process. Your feelings are very normal.

The presence of a new baby *always* modifies the interactions in a family. With the first child, husband and wife each add the role of "parent" to their identity. A second or additional child affects the "rank" of every other member of the family. Both parents are involved in these challenging adjustments and each person in the family is touched by this pregnancy.

You, a Wife

You're pregnant but hadn't planned to be. Even if your husband is the most encouraging person and is pleased and excited about this baby, you may have profound misgivings.

Career Considerations

You may be employed in a position or profession which you enjoy and wish to continue. Your career plans may not have included this child, but the fact is you *do* have a baby. If you and your husband are both in total agreement that you do not want this child, relinquishing it for adoption is an available choice. However, if this conception is the fruit of loving intercourse and/or if your husband has any positive feelings about this baby, your preference for your career may ultimately be at the expense of your marriage relationship. A workable solution may be to interrupt your career for a few years and return to it at a later date. Your decision will reflect your priorities and must be a decision with which you can live.

Fears and Concerns

The pregnancy-related problems of a married woman can have a variety of causes. You may have had a difficult previous pregnancy and have reason to be fearful. Your doctor may not be very sympathetic or you may not be comfortable with him. If you cannot or do not wish to change doctors, attempt to discuss your concerns with him. Early and regular prenatal care can lessen the severity of the other difficulties. Ask your doctor about any and all recent technological (and natural) improvements in prenatal care that you may have heard of. Medical knowledge is accumulating so rapidly that even if your now youngest child is very young, medical science has improved since its birth. There are alternative modes of childbirth; perhaps one of these may alleviate your pain and anxiety. Nearly every city has some form of childbirth education association, a good source of information for you.

Perhaps information is not your need but

rather you simply want to find someone with whom you can just talk. Groups such as Pregnancy Aid and Birthright exist to help *all* pregnant women, not only those who might be considering or experiencing pressure to have an abortion. Many of the trained volunteers in these organizations have children and will readily empathize with your emotions and concerns.

You, an Older Woman

If you are over thirty-five you might be reacting to the stories you have heard about the difficulties of an older woman bearing a child and about the increased possibility of older women giving birth to a physically or mentally impaired child. The risk of bearing a handicapped child does rise with the age of the mother. However, consider that the most common affliction, Downs Syndrome, often called Mongolism, affects approximately two percent of the babies born to over-forty mothers. This figure also says that ninety-eight percent are *not* afflicted. Of the children born with Downs Syndrome, a *small* percentage are profoundly retarded, while most are trainable and educable. Families with a Downs Syndrome child often relate that it was *this* child who united the family and taught other members the meaning of love. To learn to love is a gift!

Doctors in most genetics counseling programs report that the majority of parents who come for consultation do so not to destroy the child but to plan for the child and for the total family if their child should have a handicap. In almost every community there is help available today for both the afflicted person and for the parents. Throughout society disabled persons are leading happy, productive lives.

Your Lost Freedom

Perhaps your youngest child has just entered school and you had dreams of your new "freedom." Now you are pregnant. It is the "youngest child" who is often responsible for keeping the parents vital, active, and interesting individuals. This new baby will help adolescents in the family keep a perspective on their own maturing sexuality. It may be that this new baby will give you and your family a new freedom rooted in a fresh outlook on life.

Social Pressure

If you already have at least two children you may be aware of innuendoes about responsibility, overpopulation, and availability of resources. Among certain groups such pressure may be very great.

There is developing an awareness that it is not so much the number of people, as it is the distribution of available goods and the exploitation of natural resources that is the major problem. However, at present there is great social pressure for you to have an abortion. It can be helpful to know that among those who suffer the most damaging effects of abortion are women who have a history of depression (or attempted suicide), those who later realize that the aborted "blob" that they were told about was, in fact, a human life. The sense of relief after an abortion is short-lived and is quickly followed by the hardest kind of grief—that which feels a "guilt" or responsibility for the death.

This child, be it your first, fifth or fifteenth, is a uniquely gifted individual who will add a beauty to the world that no one else can contribute. This child will give to you a love that would otherwise be forever absent from your life.

Legally, you have the total jurisdiction over this child's right to birth. Practically, your choice of life for this baby is of great significance for your husband.

The Husband

For all the legal obligations that a father has, he does not have a legal right to protect the life of his unborn child. The young husband who returned home from work and discovered the dead body of his wife lying on the bathroom floor had not even known that she was pregnant. Her "safe, legal" abortion had caused a fatal hemorrhage.

The emotions of a man when he learns of his wife's pregnancy may be as complex as hers. A new father-to-be has a mixture of excitement and anxiety, pride and fear, and a sense of awe at being a part of the creation of a new life. A man whose wife has previously had a dangerous pregnancy and labor may panic at the thought of possibly losing the woman whom he loves while simultaneously knowing how much he cherishes his children. If he insisted on having intercourse at a time when his wife preferred not to, he may have some regret and guilt stirring within. Pinched finances may loom big in his mind, as he worries about how to feed, clothe, and educate this child. Finally, a man who suspects that this baby is not his child may rage at his wife's infidelity.

The quality of the relationship between husband and wife is the most vital factor in managing pregnancy. Pregnancy becomes a spotlight calling attention to feelings and values which may have gone unnoticed. Honest, open, and loving communication is essential to overcoming any gaps that the pregnancy might uncover in a relationship. If there is a solid basis of respect, trust, and mutual gentle tenderness, there is *no* insoluble problem. If this foundation is missing, have the courage to seek some form of family counseling.

Some husbands literally hide behind their legal powerlessness. When a wife indicates that she is thinking about abortion, a man may express no opinion or assure her that whatever she decides is acceptable to him. She may be looking to him to stop her, to affirm her, to convey his confidence that they can manage, and to prove that he is truly *with* her and loves their child. He may be greatly disillusioned with her when he realizes that she has ended the life of their child. He may also experience anger or disgust with himself for having so little courage to speak out and at least try to give her some help and encouragement. The marriage relationship suffers nearly irreparable damage. And it could have been different! Only profound honesty and forgiveness can heal such pain.

Another Man's Child

One pregnant wife experienced horrendous mental anguish knowing that the only man with whom she had had intercourse was her husband who was convinced that a childhood illness had left him permanently sterile. Time and maturity had somehow restored a degree of fertility. His initial refusal to be examined, his accusations, and his own smug sense of self-righteousness nearly destroyed his wife. Finally admitting that there was nothing in his wife's past that would give any indication that she might have been unfaithful, he agreed to submit to medical tests. Much counseling and healing was needed to begin to restore that marital relationship. In another case, the man had had a vasectomy only to discover that some surgeries do fail!

If it is suspected that the baby is not the husband's, it is important to ascertain the *facts* with as much sensitivity as possible. There is a prayer: "Lord keep my words sweet and tender; tomorrow I may have to eat them." How true this is for all of us when we are in distress.

Suppose that this is another man's child. It is important that you both analyze the reasons for the encounter which caused the pregnancy. Was it a one-time event? Is your marriage "dead"? Do you, as husband, to any extent share the blame—have your social or working habits left your wife alone too much and too long? Have you met her needs for affection, communication, and companionship? What are your drinking patterns? Have you ever been unfaithful, yet been forgiven by her?

Whatever the answers, the situation demands marriage counseling. No matter what your final decision, only honesty and gentleness will ease your mutual suffering. Your marriage can be rebuilt; love can overcome all.

It would require an entire volume to discuss whether such a baby should be kept or released for adoption. The baby could be given the same consideration as the offspring of a previous marriage or a child of an unwed mother. A man would automatically accept these children of another man when he marries the mother. On the other hand, if there is danger that the continued presence of this child will keep the wounds open and breed resentment, perhaps adoption is your solution. Obviously, extended counseling is essential for a life-giving decision for everyone concerned.

We Can't Afford a Baby

How does a couple determine if they can afford a baby? The wealthy family of the nineteen-year-old woman mentioned in the first chapter was truly poverty-stricken in an almost hopeless way in terms of the values they embraced. Money cannot guarantee good parenting. Often the children of the wealthy are sad and very lonely. The best things in life are still free. As a child once said, "We aren't poor. We just don't have any money."

The poverty that results "only" from a lack of money is solvable. Perhaps you need help in budgeting from your local social services office. You may be eligible for a low-interest loan from a city or county program. Many churches and fraternal organizations have temporary help available. The person who is able and willing to work and who has honestly sought a job (or better paying work) is certainly justified in applying for public assistance. A pride that would choose to destroy the life of one's own rather than to seek help is a sad kind of "pride." Your local Birthright, Pregnancy Aid, or Lifeline can steer you to many available resources.

If the financial problem is so great that, by the time the baby is born, you are still unable to find a satisfactory solution, you could consider placing the child in a temporary foster home or releasing it for adoption. I do not propose this as an *easy* answer. I do know that you can have life-long peace of mind knowing that you made it possible for a human being to live. Some parents who have placed their baby for adoption found it necessary to "inform" family and friends that the child died at birth. Others have been able to relate that, because of their circumstances, they were not able to keep the child but that they did love it enough to give it the best they could—life and a home. Can any parent do more?

Your Other Children

A mother of one child marvelled at her neighbor who has four children. "How do you ever do it?" she asked one day. "My Bobby takes all my time."

Wisely her friend replied, "That is all that my four take."

How many children are too many?

Perhaps you could not or would not wish for six more, but can you squeeze things somewhat so that this *one* will fit?

He was the youngest of seven—and his mother *did not want* this baby. She planned an abortion. An aunt intervened and the great Arthur Rubinstein was born. His family did find room for him.

Too often parents act within the family as if they had to do everything. Not surprisingly, they often feel overwhelmed by the burden and convey negative feelings toward their children, who then feel unwanted and unloved. Having no essential tasks in the family, a child senses that if he dies he will not even be missed. Being a nothing is so painful—teens (and adults) can and do try to anesthetize themselves with sex, drugs, alcohol, reckless driving, hard rock, running away, and ultimately, suicide.

What a contrast this is to those families in which every person is, in some way, making an important contribution. Children enjoy work tasks that are suitable to their abilities and attention spans. Parents should not even try to run the family alone.

Children delight in sharing information, in playing together,and in exploring with others the wonder of their world. Older children can teach the younger, and the younger can help the older. A task shared with a parent is good for both. One family member can be responsible for the day's prayer at meals; another might have to find a "joke for the day." One family rotates the daily task of discovering something of beauty to share.

Perhaps your children are all too young to help, there may be serious illness that demands your time, or you may lack homemaking skills. Some young parents have never learned cooking, house cleaning, home maintenance and the art of minor repairs because their parents did not let them help when they were children. Most social service programs have a home-makers service through which someone can come to your home and, for three or six months, work with you to teach you the skills you need. Then you can manage on your own. Most public school systems have free or low-cost adult and continuing education programs through which you can learn and enjoy yourself at the same time. Your new knowledge may help you to get a better paying job and your new skills may lessen your living costs.

How many children are too many? By taking the time to plan and to learn, you can welcome this child into your family.

Are you concerned about what your other children will think of your pregnancy? Your children are already thinking. Their hearts and minds have antennas quite receptive to the signals in the tone of your voice. They sense your acceptance or rejection of them as reflected from your words about this baby.

If your children have seen caring and affection between you and your spouse, they will know that having a baby is a natural part of family life. Your adolescents will know that "old-timers" can have romance in their lives, and that married life can get better through the years. Your children will learn that sex is not just a game and a fun thing to do. Having your children sense your love and responsibility for each other is worth any fifty lectures which you could give them.

In addition, all the marvels of creation to which you have tried to introduce them pale before the magnitude of this greatest wonder of all

—the gift of new life! Children's sense of awe in knowing of your pregnancy is a beautiful thing. Consider what their inner reaction would be if they were to learn that you are considering an abortion. You are carrying their brother or sister. How much do you care about them if you could have an abortion is a natural question for children to raise. Even if you should have an abortion without the children knowing about it, your relationship with them will never be the same. Each child will remind you of the baby you did not bring home; your spontaneous delight in another's baby will not be the same; you will touch and hug your own in a changed way which they will detect. What a risk, what stakes to gamble!

The Divorced or Widowed Woman

The woman who is widowed but is carrying her husband's child has, along with her grief for her husband and her anxiety about the birth, the peace of knowing that her husband does live on in their child.

For the woman whose pregnancy could not be by her late husband, the problem is compounded. Her other children, however, can understand loneliness, for they too are missing their father. They can accept an honest explanation when it is set in the context of grief and aloneness.

The woman who is divorced and is carrying her former husband's child must carefully analyze her feelings lest the child eventually experience the brunt of her emotions about her husband, their marriage, and the divorce. Much may depend on how extensive a network of emotional support she has from other people.

Regardless of your situation or the circumstances of the unplanned pregnancy, it is always advisable when pregnancy is a problem to seek the help of a counselor or a social worker as you decide your own future and that of your baby.

CHAPTER 4

Choosing an Alternative

There are many reasons of the *head* and of the *heart* for making a decision. Both are real and both are important. Part of your decision-making process must be your realization of which is which. *The reasons of the head will still be valid when the feelings fade.* A common danger is to form the conclusion first and then seek to justify it. This, of course, is not decision making. Remember that there are no easy answers and every choice is imperfect. A good decision is the one which will solve more problems than it causes and which, *in the long run,* will be most livable. No major decision should *ever* be made when a person is in a state of real depression, because our feelings color our view of reality. It is always better to wait than to rush into a choice that cannot succeed.

You will have to live the rest of your life

with whatever you choose. Other people can and should give you information and suggestions. As much as possible, the father of the baby should be part of the process. Those who are close to you want you to be happy now and after the crisis is over. Outsiders who have more experience and a wider perspective can tell you much that neither you nor your family could know. It is important that you listen and hear, with your heart and with your head. Afterwards, when you have "second thoughts" you must be able to reinforce yourself with the reasons upon which you based your decision, and then be at peace.

Your first decision concerns the life of the baby. If you have considered abortion, the information in the previous chapters will lead you to reject this action. Having made this decision, you must now focus on what is best for the future of you and your baby.

Those of you who are married will probably keep and welcome the child. However, if the baby's father is not your husband, you should at least consider adoption. There is danger that the continued presence of the child will be a constant source of resentment and anger. Both the child and the marriage will be victims. This must be a joint decision made with much love and understanding of each other's feelings. Further, if the financial and other stresses which made your pregnancy a problem in the first place are not in the process of resolution, even if the child is conceived of the marriage, adoption or temporary placement with your relatives can be a reasonable option. (Perhaps the society which, in ten years, changed abortion from a "heinous crime against humanity" into a "respectable personal choice" can someday accept a married couple's release of a baby for adoption as having its own respectability.)

Marriage

There was a time when in a case of the pregnancy of an unwed woman there was only one honorable thing to do. Marriage was hastily arranged and "they lived happily ever after." Not always did they live "happily" nor do they today. A second mistake cannot correct or erase a first mistake. Currently between 70 and 75% of teen marriages end in divorce, and when pregnancy is *the* reason for the marriage, the failure rate is nearly 90%. There are many causes for this predictable outcome. The unwed man or woman considering marriage as a "solution" to an unplanned pregnancy should carefully consider the following points.

1. There are three major transitions in the lives of most people. They are the changes from:

adolescence to adulthood
single life to married life
nonparenthood to parenthood.

Each development requires time in itself and the completion of the previous stage. In a teenage marriage where pregnancy is involved, you must make *all* of these transitions *at one time.* Over and above handling these role changes, you must complete the tasks of normal psychological development. You must discover who you are, and then accept and learn to like your total self in a profound, mature, and joyous way. You need to set the goals and adopt the life-values which will guide your adult life. This *inner growth cannot be hastened* and its absence accounts for many of the adjustment problems a couple faces in their first ten years of marriage.

Do I know and like myself?

Can I function out of my own inner values and convictions?

What are my real goals in life?

Is my boyfriend (or girlfriend) a mature adult?

2. Often a pregnancy is subconsciously wanted or planned to make possible an escape from the current home situation. Marriage, however, demands a positive commitment and it cannot be seen as an escape from anything. We take ourselves with us wherever we go, and exchanging one set of problems for another set really does not solve much.

Why did I get pregnant?

Why do I want to get married?

What problems will I take with me into a marriage?

3. You and/or your partner may not have discovered and accepted who you are and are therefore not ready to make a marriage commitment. You may be incapable of discovering and accepting the other as a person. We do not expect a one-year-old to read; we should not require psychological tasks that are beyond our own or another's stage of development. Not only is it unfair; it may actually hinder necessary growth.

Am I capable of self-giving and responsibility?

Is my boy (or girl) friend capable of mature giving?

4. When sexual activity becomes a part of an unmarried couple's relationship, it often arrests the finding and nurturing of common interests, values, and communication skills upon which a life together depends.

What values and interests do we share?

What values and interests can we develop?

In what ways do we communicate?

How deeply do we communicate?

What do we have going for us besides "sex"?

5. The reality of married life does not fit the myths and illusions which the media present about marriage. While love is blind, marriage is an eye-opener.

What have you experienced in your own families that you want in your marriage?

What strengths do you see in each other?

What weaknesses do you see?

How do you deal with the petty annoyances caused by the people you live with now?

How "big" are "little" things when *you* do them? When someone else does them?

6. One or both of you may have unresolved feelings of resentment toward the other, or a sense of personal guilt in regard to the pregnancy. "Forgive and start over" is a basic rule for successful living and an absolute necessity in marriage.

How much do either of you blame the other?

Have you taken your resentment or anger out on anyone else? Might you transfer that resentment to your baby?

7. Is your income inadequate for the needs of an instant family? It is likely that you will both need to cut back on the style of living to which you are accustomed. Money difficulties can often threaten a good, mature marriage in which there is already a proven ability to sacrifice. If the strength to postpone the satisfaction of wants is not present in both partners, the challenge is all the greater. Most community social service programs have a budget specialist. This is the person to see *while* you are in the decision-making process.

Can you improvise when you must?

Can you do without conveniences and luxuries?

Can you enjoy free or inexpensive entertainment?

Is your income adequate in relation to the real cost-of-living in your locality?

8. Problems of adjustment arise in every marriage and family. When problems arise in a "forced" marriage the baby can easily become, at least subconsciously, an object of blame and resentment: "If it wasn't for you, we wouldn't have had to get married." Under severe stress, even good parents may abuse their children. For every instance of physical abuse there may be as many as twenty of psychological abuse. Even if there is "only" a lack of warmth and affection for the child, the damage can be serious and permanent. We tend to parent as we have been parented. If you are dissatisfied with your relationship with your own parents, you would do well to enter some parenting education program or to read as much about child development as you can. It would be good if you had or could have some actual experience in caring for children.

How much do you know about child care and development?

How gentle and patient can you be?

Can you adjust to a child's time schedule?

Can you communicate, nonverbally as well as with words, to infants, to babies, to toddlers?

9. It is important to consider the attitudes of both sets of parents, for the support of parents and in-laws increases the likelihood of a marriage being successful. Grandparents have little trouble accepting their grandchild, but often they never admit or come to terms with their resentment toward "that boy" (or girl) who "got my little girl (or son) in trouble."

Do you like and respect your future in-laws?

How do they feel about you?

Do your parents like and respect your future partner? How does he (or she) relate to your parents?

How do the future grandparents relate to their other grandchildren?

How do they talk about other young people who have been in this situation?

Are you strong enough to build your marriage in spite of opposition or interference from parents and in-laws?

Can you understand and love your parents in the face of these difficulties?

It is a simple fact that despite the odds against the marriage lasting, many couples do marry to solve an out-of-wedlock pregnancy. What then?

The parents of the young couple may find themselves in an awkward predicament. They may see marriage as the solution, "for the sake of the baby," and yet know that the marriage has only a slim chance of lasting. They may find themselves unable to fully accept their child's future spouse. If both or either of the young people have reservations, the parents must see their honesty as honorable and respectable. What point is there in rushing the decision or the ceremony? Whether the baby is born within nine months after the wedding or sometime before the ceremony will not really make that much difference in the long run.* The opinion of relatives and friends is of far less importance than the stability and success of the marriage. Parents should never force a wedding; unless each partner is psychologically free there cannot be a true marriage.

It may be the young couple that is insistent. In this case, it is counterproductive to try to forbid the wedding. A workable approach may be for both sets of parents with their children to enter into a reality-oriented counseling process with the assistance of a counselor, social worker, or member of the clergy. In this way the feelings of all can be worked through in an adult manner. Counseling may lead to a decision not to marry. If the opposite is true, the counseling process will have enhanced the chances for lasting happiness and satisfaction in the marriage.

*State laws vary as to what can be on the baby's birth certificate. Consult your social worker for this information.

If the young couple decides to marry, their parents again face an apparent contradiction. The couple need independence and the opportunity to make their marriage succeed—to grow, to learn, to laugh, to accomplish, to fail, to cry, to forgive. They require some distance and much privacy. On the other hand, they need their parents' loving concern and emotional support, especially since the baby may be born during the first crucial months of adjustment. It takes much prudence and great sensitivity for parents to work out their role in their child's marriage.

Perhaps the most difficult part of any marriage is the adjustment to countless little things and to the unexpected. Situations will arise that no one could have predicted—you will have to deal with them in loving honesty as they arise. Feelings will surface in unexpected ways. By talking through unexpected situations and feelings as they arise, you can successfully cope. While the odds are against your marriage succeeding, you need not be overcome by the difficulties. With your own love and commitment, with the support of others, and with serious preparation your marriage can be permanent.

* * * * *

The situation is somewhat different for an older couple particularly if they were already planning to be married. There are different but equally important considerations that must be resolved: Does the pregnancy change the attitude or plans of either partner? Has this unexpected development highlighted personality traits in yourself or your partner that cause either of you to have second thoughts about marriage? Was the relationship getting shaky and was pregnancy seen as a way of salvaging something from it before it completely ended? An intensive and honest re-evaluation of your relationship before the wedding can reduce second-guessing during the marriage.

* * * * *

Whatever the circumstances in which marriage is considered, ultimately the decision should solve more problems than it creates. The wedding is not the marriage; passion is not love. Only sacrificial love and hard work have ever made a marriage. Unless you have a solid foundation of shared beliefs and values, common interests, great trust and respect, the marriage will probably fail. Divorce is always a trauma for both the woman and the man. Being rejected or living with a sense of failure is very painful. The breakup of a family is always the hardest on the child or children and may do them more damage than if they were raised by a single parent or were released for adoption.

Single Parenting

The ability to put another person's concerns ahead of your own is a sign of being an adult. It takes a person with a mature self-image to consider the needs of another over his or her own. While your needs and dreams are important, those of your baby must be your first concern. Counseling can help you attain the level of self-appreciation and maturity needed not to be threatened by placing your baby's needs first. Interestingly enough, the choice that is best for your baby is also the decision that, in the long run, is best for you.

Every child has a right to be raised by a mature parent. There are serious reasons for insisting that adults, not children, should be raising children. In the world of reality there are heavy stresses which often overwhelm even the most loving, caring parent. It sometimes happens that a woman who was confident that she could raise her child alone is later on overcome by stress and ends up placing the baby for adoption. Such children bear the double scar of the results of their parents' stress and of the anguish of separation which they are too young to understand. Often they feel they have been sent away because they have been "bad" and a burden of guilt then follows them through life.

Social agencies are too often treating young victims of physical and psychological abuse, as well as single parents who have been damaged even as they did the abusing. So often, such a parent is a mother who was so very sure that she would be the perfect parent and never hurt her child in any way. Most of these parents are good people, and under normal conditions they would never hurt anyone. They were simply unable to cope with the demands of single-parenting.

You can be helped to understand the reality of single parenting by reading some of the helpful material on the subject. Your librarian will help you locate books on the general topic or particular aspects. Particularly valuable for you is Chapter Two, "The Importance of Being Honest," in Carole Klein's book, *The Single Parent Experience*. Read, think, reread. Talk it over with your parents and your counselor. Talk over *all* the issues on both sides of this decision. Many agencies have valuable rap sessions for new and prospective single parents. Listening to other single parents sharing their problems, expressing feelings, and asking questions can be very helpful to you.

As you read and discuss, your challenge is to be honest and to listen. Later you can argue for one side or the other; right now, openness to all insights is most important in answering these questions:

What are my real and deep reasons for wanting to keep my baby?

What do I know about babies? About toddlers? Do I know how to take care of a sick baby?

Can I afford this child? Can I manage money?

Who will be the primary care-giver for my baby?

What needs will my baby have? Can I fill them?

What needs do I have?

What resources will be available to both of us?

Parenting Is Serious Business

Parenting is a serious undertaking. Having a baby takes nine months; parenting lasts a lifetime. Recently numerous books about mothering, fathering, and parenting have been published. They all testify to the difficulties that all parents face in the sacred task of nurturing a child entrusted to them. No one *owns* a child. A parent is *for* the child. While a parent may have some of her or his own needs met by a child, this is only a side result, a by-product, of being a parent. A child should be kept or adopted for the sake of meeting the child's needs, and never for the sake of the parents, to hold a marriage together, or to prove a point.

Earlier in this book you were asked to analyze the reasons why you became pregnant. Now you must explore your real, deep, inner reasons why you would keep your baby. Do you like children? Do you enjoy child-centered activities? Can you accept this unique human being and encourage his or her development and interests? Can you rejoice whether this child is a boy or girl? Have you resolved any negative or angry feelings you have for the baby's father or for men in general? Daughters of single mothers often grow up disliking themselves as women and hating men. A son may be expected to be the "man of the family" and not have a chance to be a normal little boy. You do not want to catch yourself saying in anger to your child "You are just like your father." Can you balance discipline and freedom in your own life? Can you develop both in a child? On days when you feel resentful and trapped, can you maintain an even composure? How will you answer your child's inevitable question, "Why don't I have a daddy?"

It has been said that children need human parents—not perfect parents. If you are imagining yourself raising a child as you wish you had been raised, you may be placing unreal and damaging demands on your baby. (Your baby must be a "good" baby so people will see that you are a "good" parent.) Unrealistic expectations put pressures on a parent, and these stresses eventually affect the child. In contrast, good parenting requires the ability to relax, to resist attempting to meet someone else's expectations. How else can you enjoy your child and also rejoice in yourself as a parent? Parenting, like all the other beautiful things of life, is meant to be a joy!

Parenting is a demanding commitment. It makes demands on both parents. A mother and father can develop a rhythm of responsibility. Neither parent has to feel the full twenty-four-hour burden. For you as a single parent the total responsibility will be on your shoulders—for eighteen years. Your baby will be an infant for only a few months. Very soon you will have a teething, crying, getting-into-everything, question-asking, "NO"-saying individual. You might profit from half-a-day of just strolling through some stores to observe the mothers and children whom you see there. Mentally put yourself in the mothers' shoes. Do they fit?

What experiences have you already had with children? Your age, the size family from which you come, the times you have tended children, will all make an important difference for you. Do you know what to do or where to find answers if your baby has an earache at 2:30 AM? (Babies and children seldom get sick at convenient times.) How do you baby-proof a house or apartment? What makes a toy safe or unsafe? How do you comfort a baby awakened and scared by a storm, or who is screaming and cannot tell you what it wants or where it hurts? Are you aware of what a child can do at certain stages of growth? Much abuse occurs when the parent is impatient for a child to do something that it just is not able to do.

Because raising another human being places such heavy burdens on a parent, you will have to read, study, discuss, listen, and learn a great deal. Here you can benefit from the single parent rap sessions referred to earlier. They are often the only occasion when a single mother can express her true feelings. Talking can be a safety valve so that pressures do not build up and lead to abuse. You can also anticipate the great joy it is to learn from a child, if you are open to the awe and wonder to which a child may lead you. You may delight in watching an ant crawling in the grass, in the mystery of sand (and mud), and in the pleasure of splashing water at a lake (or all over the bathroom). You will need to be ready to let go in a light-hearted rejoicing that will make both of you glad to be alive and to have each other.

The issues of money, where you will live, and who will care for your baby are interrelated. Your age, education, and skills will make a great difference in the type of work available to you and in your earning power.

If, because of your age, you continue living with your parents, you may find that they are paying for much that you and your baby need. Payment of money usually results in control—who will make the decisions for you and your baby? Will you still be a "child" or can you be an adult woman in your parents' home? Will your child be more oriented to your mother than to you? A child needs the security of knowing upon whom he or she can depend to be there when there is a need, or a hurt, or something nice to share. If there is any friction between you and your parents it will produce tension and that may affect your child. On the other hand, if during this crisis time while you have waited for your child's birth, you and your parents have worked through your conflicts or have at least come to understand and trust each other more, your parents' home could be a very secure place for both the baby and you.

An older, working mother has a different set of questions. Who will care for your baby while you are working? Whatever option you choose—day-care, a sitter who comes into your home or one who cares for children in her own home, a relative—your baby has to adjust to someone besides yourself. More and more psychologists are coming back to the "old-fashioned" idea that a young child needs the continued presence of its parent. While you may read that "it's not the amount of time that you spend with your child that matters but rather the quality of the time," you must remember that a child needs *both,* a great amount of time and your *best* time. The hours before work and the tired hours afterwards are not the best time for most people. The working mother may have one advantage that the nonworking, living-alone parent does not have: adult company and conversation during the day. She is able to experience a sense of doing something "worthwhile." Although caring for a child is tremendously important, it does not always *feel* significant.

Single Parent Needs

Should you choose to live alone with your child and not work, you will need to arrange some time when you are in touch with other adults. Loneliness is the most common complaint of the single mother. Although she loves her child and is a good mother, she needs the input of ideas and two-way communication. Married parents can share, cry, and laugh together over the first words and the enjoyable antics of their child—the single mother may have no one with whom to share these moments.

One problem which all single parents have in common is whether and how to have a social life. A recent study showed that six years after the birth of their first child, fifty percent of single parents were still single. Being a single parent complicates the effort to form friendships and significant relationships particularly with the opposite sex. Loneliness is a common condition of the single parent. Unless the child has playmates its own age, loneliness will also be a problem for the child. Some "only children" report that they enjoyed being an "only," but there are very many that would testify to the desolation of growing up alone.

Among single parents there are few who have sufficient money to fulfill their dreams. Rents are soaring; the expenses of a car are draining budgets; costs for everything from food to doing laundry are reaching critical limits for many people. The single parent can often benefit from help in budgeting.

In addition to material things, you and your child have other needs. Your child should be introduced to books, to sports, to toys with which the imagination can run free, to music and art, to animals and to growing things—to the world. You, too, deserve a world of ever-widening interests. You can take advantage of the many free and inexpensive activities in your community. Your public library can be a source of information about what is available. The more your funds are limited, the more you need your library for books, magazines, records, even pictures on your walls. Some libraries have children's story hours, films, and a host of other offerings. Librarians like nothing better than to have their materials used and their activities attended, all of which are free!

You can also utilize the resources of the agency that is helping or has helped you in your pregnancy. The more resourceful you become the better you will feel about yourself; this alive you is the best gift you can give your child.

Adoption

In many ways adoption may be the most difficult course of action for you to consider. Like the other options, it is best to explore it carefully with the help of others. Your parents and the baby's father should definitely be part of the counseling process.

Your thoughts about adoption may reflect many generally accepted but inaccurate ideas. Up-to-date information is critical if you are to make a well-thought-out decision.

The Adoption Process

Procedures for adoption are very different today from what they were as recently as ten years ago. No longer is adoption considered an automatic or simple answer to an unplanned pregnancy. You do have a choice, and the final decision is *yours,* both by your right as a mother and by law. Your counselor will help you to understand your rights, to explore both your *head* reasons and your *heart* reasons for your possible choices, and help you to plan realistically how you will carry out your decision. The counselor who has come to know you, your abilities and your resources, *may* feel very strongly that a certain choice is the best one for you to make and may feel that you are mature enough to listen to the reasons why such seems to be the best course. The counselor may even attempt to persuade you to a particular course of action. In the end, however, the decision is *yours*—yours to make and yours to *live.*

During counseling sessions you can ask any question that comes to your mind. Your questions are a sign that you are thinking ahead, admitting your feelings, and honestly seeking what is best for you and your baby. Your counselor can only respond to your questions and meet your needs if you ask. Having no questions may signify that you are not being realistic and that you are too immature to be a good parent if you do choose to keep the baby. The only "dumb question" is the one you do not ask. It may be the first time *you* asked this question, but it most certainly will not be the first time the counselor has heard it.

In general, today's adoption procedures encourage the new mother not only to see her baby but to hold it and to give him or her a name. She may be given a picture of the baby. She may also prepare a letter and/or gift that the adoptive parents can give the child when he or she is old enough to wonder why he or she was released for adoption. It is acceptable for you to tell your counselor if there is any particular type of mother and/or father and home which you would like your baby to have. Today most adoption agencies tell the natural mother a great deal of nonidentifying information about the adoptive parents.

After You Release the Baby

If you release your baby for adoption, it is natural that you will live with many on-going questions. You will wonder about how the child is growing and getting along in school, if he or she has many friends, what hobbies and interests the child has, and if your child ever thinks of you. Birthdays and holidays will always have a special significance and be a time of unanswered wondering.

If you do decide to release your baby for adoption, you give up only your legal rights; you do not give up your feelings of love for your child or your sadness because your baby is no longer with you. You will always have a place in your heart and in your prayers for this child. There will be times of sadness and of tears. In the midst of all these thoughts you will, however, have a conviction: *that you gave primary consideration to your baby's best interest and acted with great courage and love.* Your child can grow up with the conviction that somewhere there is a woman who *cared very much.*

Because you have cared so much and because there will be an emptiness, very keen at first, you must expect to experience a sense of loss and grief. The "experts" tell us that two years is the average duration for grieving and that, even after this length of time, there may be an abiding sense of loss. On those days when anger, depression, sadness, and loneliness come, know that such feelings are normal. It will help considerably to talk about the feelings and thoughts you are having. At the same time, it will help if you have creative and enjoyable personal growth interests and activities to which you can turn. Your maturity will manifest itself as you find a balance somewhere between never and always talking about your experience and about the baby. (It is better to talk too much than not to talk enough, however, when a person is working through grief.) Seek to find a midpoint between inactivity and losing yourself in hyperactivism.

Many women who release a child for adoption consider the act of signing the final papers as the end of the process and they discontinue contact with their counselor. However, this person who now knows you very well could be a great help at this time. During pregnancy both you and the counselor were faced with a deadline for making decisions about the pregnancy. Now together you can, with less pressure, deal with your ongoing feelings and growth, and with the root issues that surfaced as you were reading Chapter One. Counselors have often indicated that they wished there would be further opportunity to continue but that the "exhaustion" of labor, delivery, and release causes many women to stop coming. It would be very worthwhile to consider meeting with your counselor, at least once within three months after the final papers are signed.

Some Difficulties

There are four additional sources of stress at the time of the adoption decision for you to consider. The first is the pressure from your parents (or the baby's father) for you to keep the baby. It is very hard for your parents, especially if this is their first grandchild, to know that you are considering adoption. As much as you love your parents (or as difficult as your relationship with them may be), *you* are the person who will have to live with this decision for the rest of your life.

A second source of stress may be pressure from your friends. They are thinking only of a cuddly and lovable baby—you are thinking of a distinct human being who will grow up, have needs and a claim on your life for eighteen years. *You* are the one who will walk the floors at night, have little social life, and have all the problems of the single parent.

Thirdly, the adoption identity movement —the search by birth parents for the children they released for adoption, and the efforts of adopted children to discover their roots—can be a source of stress. The fact that *some* adoptees are searching for their birth parents could make you think that an adopted person is unhappy. Not so! *Many* adoptees are *not* searching. Of those who are, most are reacting to the fact that, in their case *no* information about their origin was communicated. They are men and women who have a normal curiosity about their ethnic background and their medical history. Some would like to establish contact with their birth parents, but most recognize and appreciate the fact that their birth parents have had a chance to start over and to rebuild their lives. Most adoptees will conclude: "If my birth parents cared enough about me to make the sacrifice they did, then I care enough about them to respect their wishes about a reunion." The states which do have "open records" legislation have structured their procedures to respect the rights and wishes of both the birth parents and the adoptee, and require mutual agreement before identifying information is released or contact is arranged.

Whether you will have or want a reunion with your child eighteen years in the future is not an issue which you must decide now. Know that this may be a possibility, then let the matter rest until the time comes and deal with it at that time.

A fourth source of stress is the *normal* conflict between your natural desire that this baby should be part of your life and your natural fears and questions about your ability to parent the baby as he or she deserves. Do not be surprised if, during your pregnancy, you waver back and forth in your decision. The hardest moments may well be immediately after the baby's birth when you have seen, held, and loved your child. Nurses and doctors have been known to make very thoughtless remarks. Your *head* reasons will have to be very strong, especially at this time.

Adoption will not be easy and you will carry painful memories with you. However, adoption is the choice which does give you a chance to start over, and for you this may well be the greatest advantage that releasing the baby will have.

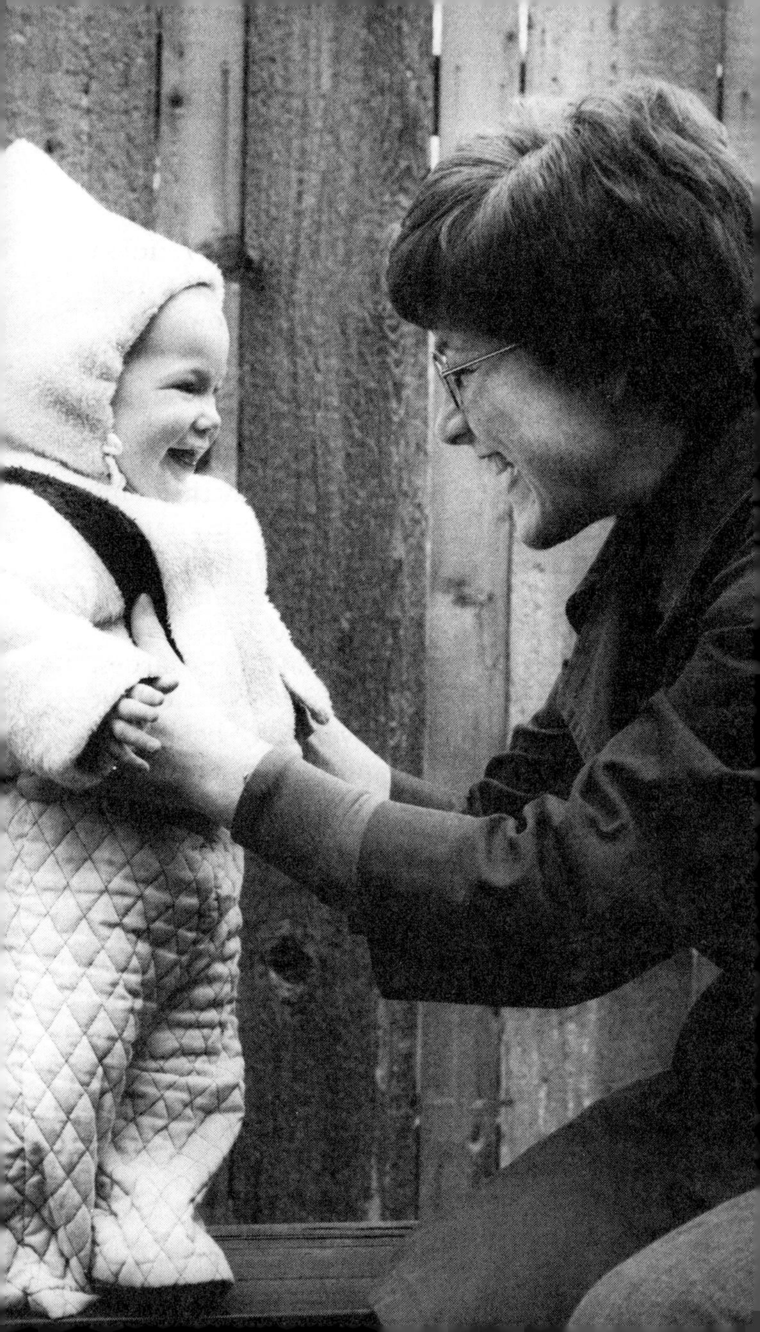

Conclusion

This book, and especially this last chapter, has not been easy for you to read—you may now have many more questions than when you began.

If you—or the woman whom you want to help—have simply read these pages on your own, I again encourage you to seek trained help. This is a time when it is not good to be alone. There are countless people "out there"—clergy and religious, social workers, counselors, teachers, and other professional persons. There are also dedicated, caring, trained volunteers at Birthright, Pregnancy Aid, Lifeline, and similar groups.

All of these people care very much about you. They are anxious to help. You need only to call them.

You are no longer alone.

Suggestions for Further Reading

Baars, Conrad M.D. *Born Only Once: The Miracle of Affirmation*. Chicago: Franciscan Herald Press, 1975.

Ball, John and Nancy. *Joy in Human Sexuality*. Collegeville: Liturgical Press, 1975.

Colman, Arthur and Libby. *Pregnancy: The Psychological Experience*. New York: Seabury Press, 1971.

Delahoyde, Melinda. *Fighting for Life: Defending the Newborn's Right to Live*. Ann Arbor: Servant, 1984.

Gauchat, Dorothy. *All God's Children*. New York: Ballantine, 1985.

Head, Ann. *Mr. and Mrs. Bo Jo Jones*. New York: Putnam, 1967.

Hekman, Randall J. *Justice for the Unborn.* Ann Arbor: Servant, 1984.

Ingelman-Sundberg, A. *A Child is Born: The Drama of Life before Birth.* New York: Dell Publishing Company, 1966.

Johnston, Patricia, ed. *Perspectives on a Grafted Tree: Thoughts for Those Touched by Adoption.* Fort Wayne: Perspectives Press, 1982.

Klein, Carole. *The Single Parent Experience.* New York: Avon Books, 1973.

Liley, Helen and Day, B.F. *Modern Motherhood: Pregnancy, Childbirth, and the Newborn Baby.* New York: Random House, 1969.

Losoncy, Larry. *When Your Child Needs a Hug.* St. Meinrad: Abbey Press, 1978.

Macmanus, Sheila. *The Adoption Book.* Ramsey: Paulist, 1984.

Nathanson, Bernard M.D. and Ostling, Richard. *Aborting America.* New York: Doubleday, 1979.

Powell, John S.J. *Fully Human, Fully Alive.* Niles: Argus, 1976.

Powell, John, S.J. *Abortion: The Silent Holocaust.* Niles: Argus, 1981.

Quesnell, John M.S.W. *Marriage: A Discovery Together.* Notre Dame: Fides, 1974.

Salk, Lee Ph.D. and Kramer, Rita. *How to Raise a Human Being.* New York: Warner, 1969.

Shettles, Landrum, M.D. and Rorvik, David. *Rites of Life: The Scientific Evidence for Life before Birth.* Grand Rapids: Zondervan, 1983.

Sorosky, Arthur M.D.; Baran, Annette M.S.W. and Pannor, Reuben. *The Adoption Triangle.* Garden City: Anchor Books, 1978.

Torney, John C. *Emotional Child Abuse.* Canfield: Alba, 1979.